Caring For Those With
ALZHEIMER'S
A Pastoral Approach

Caring For Those With ALZHEIMER'S A Pastoral Approach

*

JOAN D. ROBERTS

ALBA · HOUSE NEW · YORK

SOCIETY OF ST. PAUL, 2187 VICTORY BLVD., STATEN ISLAND, NEW YORK 10314

Scripture quotations from the Revised Standard Version of the Bible copyright © 1946, 1952, 1957 by Division of Christian Education of the National Council of the Churches of Christ in the United States of American.

Some of the material in this book appeared in a different form in the article "Through the Eyes of Alzheimer's: A Pastoral Approach" by Joan D. Roberts, in the November, 1989 issue of Pastoral Life *magazine, Canfield, Ohio 44406.*

Library of Congress Cataloging-in-Publication Data

Roberts, Joan D., 1953 -
    Caring for those with Alzheimer's : a postoral approach /
Joan D. Roberts.
        p.   cm.
    Includes bibliographical references.
    ISBN 0-8189-0593-X
    1. Caregivers — Religious life. 2. Alzheimer's disease —
Religous aspects — Christianity. 3. Alzheimer's disease — Patients
— Home care. 4. Church work with the terminally ill. 5. Church work
with the aged. I. Title.
B4910.9.R63 1991   90-26574
259'.4 — dc20   CIP

Designed, printed and bound in the United States of
America by the Fathers and Brothers of the
Society of St. Paul, 2187 Victory Boulevard,
Staten Island, New York 10314, as part of their
communications apostolate.

© Copyright 1991 by Joan D. Roberts

PRINTING INFORMATION:

Current Printing - first digit 1 2 3 4 5 6 7 8 9 10 11 12

Year of Current Printing - first year shown

1991	1992	1993	1994	1995	1996	1997	1998

Dedication

This book is most warmly dedicated to Maria, and to all Alzheimer's patients and caregivers. It is also dedicated in a very special way to all who have known suffering, and who try to make life a little happier and brighter for others. For all the hope and encouragement you bring — thank you!

Joan D. Roberts

Contents

Introduction ix
1. Maria 1
2. Background Information 13
3. Keeping Perspective 21
4. Listen to Your Feelings 27
5. Spirituality and the Caregiver 35
6. Psychotherapy and Pastoral Care ... 45
7. Practical Tips 51
8. Nursing Homes 57
9. A Word to Pastors 67
10. A Sample Homily 73
11. Scripture Readings 77
Suggested Readings/Resources 83

Introduction

ALZHEIMER'S DISEASE is the fourth largest killer
of American adults, after heart disease, cancer,
and stroke. It claims some 100,000 lives each
year. There may be as many as four million
people suffering from Alzheimer's nationwide
— a figure that may rise to fourteen million by
the year 2050.

Some 70% of Alzheimer's patients remain
at home, and eventually need around the clock
attention.

I wrote this little book with two purposes in
mind: to help Alzheimer's caregivers in their
duties, and to show pastors and counselors how
the needs of the caregiver can be met.

Of course, I don't pretend to give a com-
plete and exhaustive treatment of Alzheimer's
Disease and the problems it causes. This book
will have served its purpose if it gives enough
information and tips to help make the lives of
the Alzheimer's patient and the caregiver as
bearable as possible.

I know what it's like to be a caregiver of an
Alzheimer's patient. I'll share with you my story
of Maria, whom I dearly love. At this writing,

she has been progressively deteriorating from this disease in the center where she has been for over a year. "Maria," of course, is not her real name. I've changed it and the names of her family members to protect their privacy.

If it weren't for Maria, I probably would never have given a second thought to Alzheimer's Disease. I'm sure that most Alzheimer's caregivers did not expect to find themselves in this role.

I dedicate this book to Maria. For her and for all those who suffer like her, I pray that their suffering will bear as much fruit as possible. May they move us to learn about this terrible disease and to support the Alzheimer's Association and its research, so that fewer stories like theirs will be told across the land.

Joan D. Roberts

CHAPTER 1

Maria

"HER MEMORY IS BAD," he told me. We sat at the kitchen table in Maria's house. Her son Bill, who lived in the area, was looking for a female companion for his mother. At the moment, she was visiting his older brother Joe and family in Atlanta.

I was referred to him by a mutual friend, a nurse who had cared for Maria while she was briefly hospitalized. Bill was anxious to have me move in, saying that he hadn't advertised in the papers, and that I came highly recommended.

I needed another job to supplement my income, and I was experienced in dealing with elderly people. I would work in my regular job during the day, and be a companion to Maria in the evening.

I was excited about this, but very apprehensive. Maria and I had never met! I had to agree on this position without even meeting her!

Bill gave me a bit of background information. Then, still somewhat apprehensive, I said, "Well, if I'm not going to meet her before I move in, at least let me see her picture!" He smiled, and promptly produced a family album. I was *delighted* with what I saw!

The pictures showed a short Italian woman with warm brown eyes and a loving smile. She was now 69 years old. Her husband, who was with her in the pictures, had died the previous year of a sudden heart attack while they were in a park enjoying a concert. In recent years, she had lost several of her family and friends who were very dear to her. Many years ago, she had lost three daughters shortly after they were born.

Bill told me that he felt that all of these losses took a heavy toll on her and affected her memory. He also mentioned that some of her brothers lived nearby with their families, and one brother, Tom, was especially faithful in visiting her daily.

I took the job. We shook hands and agreed on the terms. Then I went home, little realizing that this was going to be one of the biggest challenges of my life thus far!

I thought that Maria would be even more nervous than I was. At least I had seen her pictures — she didn't even know what I looked like. All she was told was that a good friend of her former nurse was going to move in with her. In view of all the recent adjustments she had gone through, this was bound to be stressful for her. But of course, I reasoned, she loved and trusted her son, and so I hoped for the best for the both of us.

Within a week, I moved in. It was a little before Christmas, 1986. As I was coming up the driveway, I saw Maria in the window, and my apprehensions vanished. Her warm smile caused me to feel that I had made the right decision. I knew we were going to be good friends. That night, she showed me how she made pork chops. After we cleaned up, we talked for hours. I had brought a few things with me to spend the night, and was preparing for the big move the next day. I felt very peaceful and loved, and happily retired for the night.

Since we were initially so compatible, Maria and I quickly adjusted to life together. Her family members who lived nearby were also pleased at how things were turning out. I knew that Maria had a bad memory, but she was such a *wonderful* person, and she managed most things fairly well.

It was only gradually that I began to see things that worried me. Each day I would go to work, and Maria would cook supper early — only she made too much of the same things and reheated them night after night. I couldn't reason with her about throwing the food out, as

- 3 -

she thought it was all fresh. I forced myself to eat what I could, and tried to dispose of the rest without her knowledge.

Maria was understandably depressed about her husband's death and the approaching holidays. Surely, I thought, she was too young to be going senile. I encouraged her to cry, to let it all out, to talk — whatever she wanted. I gave her lots of affection — which was easy to do, as she was very lovable. I encouraged her to go out with me as often as possible after work to the malls or other places, so that she would be stimulated by the lights, people, and activity. She seemed to enjoy this for a while, but would revert to her depression. I also tried telling her lots of jokes, which helped to lighten the atmosphere. Maria had a wonderful laugh.

We had Bill and his family over for dinner on Christmas, and all went well. Time melted into January, 1987, and our daily routine continued.

More things began happening. Maria wanted to go to bed as soon as it was dark, and would wake up disoriented in the middle of the night. She lost the ability to tell time or read a calendar. I began to call her from work, besides leaving a note each morning, to remind her that I was at work and would be home at a certain time. But as time passed, this became less and less effective.

Maria's hygiene habits also began to suffer. She was afraid to take a bath or shower because she had forgotten the procedure, but couldn't admit it. She was constantly misplacing things, and blaming me or others for moving or taking them. She couldn't manage her money, and so that fell to me. She couldn't read much below the headlines of a paper, and would read those several times over. She also couldn't keep track of the plots of TV shows — TV became a series of meaningless images to her.

Maria began to have sudden, unusual mood swings and crying jags, and as time passed, these became more frequent. When I asked her what she was crying about, she couldn't often say what the reason was. She seemed to remember events of long ago with astounding clarity, but often couldn't remember what happened yesterday or even an hour ago.

Physically, her eyesight and hearing were excellent. But she began to be disturbed by normal, everyday noises, such as the furnace going on, or the noise a washing machine makes. One day, just as I was starting to take a shower before work, I heard her scream! My heart racing, I stopped the shower, covered myself, and went to investigate. She was in bed. "What are you screaming about?" I asked. "The shower is too noisy," she replied. I was amazed

— "I've been taking a shower every day around this time. If it bothered you, why didn't you tell me before?" She couldn't answer that, and remained silent. I nervously finished getting ready for work, and left. I was experiencing a great deal of anger and mixed emotions. It was very hard for me to work that day, and I dreaded the thought of going home. But by the time I got there, she was in a good mood and had forgotten all about what had happened that morning.

I tried to tell Bill about these things, but he always came up with excuses. I became close friends with Maria's brother Tom, who visited her daily, and with his family. They understood, and they helped me to persevere through all of this. I shared my feelings with my closest friends, who often asked, "Why don't you just leave?"

But I couldn't. Despite everything, I grew to love Maria, who — in her more lucid moments — was the most loving and gentle person you could hope to find. I would do anything in my power to avoid abandoning her. She had lost so many people already. So had I, and knew what it was like.

For her part, Maria was becoming increasingly dependent on me for every little thing. I worried about her tremendously, and called her from work whenever possible. I found it hard to concentrate on things at work. Even on my free time out, I could not get Maria off my mind. I was always thinking of what she was going through, and how I could understand her better.

It was around this time that I went to a local library and found the book, *The 36 Hour Day: A Family Guide to Caring for Persons with Alzheimer's Disease, Related Dementing Illness, and Memory Loss in Later Life*, by Nancy L. Mace and Peter V. Rabins, MD. I was riveted by the first paragraphs! The more I read, the more I recognized Maria! Halfway through the book, I felt sick to my stomach. I had to put it down and leave. The thought that Maria had this disease and would ultimately go through these changes was more than I could bear. I was terrified of what the future would bring.

With God's grace, we made it through the winter and into the spring. Maria loved flowers and gardening, and I hoped that this activity would help her. When she was working with her flowers and the results turned out well, she felt proud. I tried in every way possible to build up her confidence. She often felt inferior because she hadn't finished high school and couldn't drive. She also knew that her memory was failing, as she would struggle to find words to say what she meant. She would often call herself stupid or dumb, and I told her emphatically not to, that it wasn't her fault.

It became increasingly more heartbreaking for all of us to have to see her deteriorating step by step like that, and most nerve-wracking never knowing what to expect from one moment to the next. At times like these, one's faith is sorely tested. One's loneliness can be most excruciating! But if this is the case for a caregiver and others, imagine what it must be like for the victim!

There were days when she seemed to be doing so well that my heart was full of hope and joy. Oh, how I thanked God on those days, and on those nights when we were able to just sit and talk and understand one another. I would tell her about problems at work, for instance; she was pleased that I confided in her. She also helped me put things into perspective at times. She, like anyone, needed to be needed, perhaps more than ever before. She needed to give love, too, and I think it helped that we had two neighborhood boys who always loved to come over and ride their bikes up and down the driveway, seeking her attention.

One of my most heartwarming memories of her was caused by my vulnerability, as one day my back went out at work, and the pain was excruciating. It was next to impossible for me to stand straight. I somehow managed to drive home, wondering how we would get through this, hating to upset her. But Maria was most compassionate and most ready to help. She gave me several back rubs with ointment, and her cooking even seemed to improve for the time being. She was very understanding, and enjoyed acting out her motherly role once again. I never saw her so happy that she could be of help, and was glad that something good could come out of this.

I tried to sleep in my bed, but it was no use. I struggled to the couch, from where I could push myself up, but I could not bend over to get the blanket, so just lay there, not wanting to disturb Maria. She came shortly afterward and covered me up, acting as any mother would. For the time being, it was a relief and a comfort for me to be the one who was vulnerable. Whatever happened after that, I would never forget this, and it seemed to strengthen my resolve to stay with Maria as long as I could.

This resolve was often tested as time went on. At times she got lost in her own house, which only had one story. People would visit, like Bill, and as soon as they left, she would forget they were there. Sometimes she would eat and forget shortly after that she had eaten. One of the most horrifying things, to my mind, happened when she looked straight at me and asked when I was coming home!

I used to take her to her old neighborhood, which she seemed to enjoy, but had forgotten about as soon as we got home. At times she would say she wanted to go home, and I told her she already was, but then I knew she was thinking of her childhood home. At times she had hallucinations of children, which was very disconcerting.

One year later, in September, one of her grandsons was visiting from Atlanta. While he was there, she was talking about her mother, as she often did. She said, "Where's Mom? I haven't seen her in awhile." Her mother had been dead for several years. We tried to explain that to her, and showed her the newspaper clippings. "Why didn't anyone tell me my mother died?" was her response, as she cried bitterly. This happened several times each day after that.

Eventually her grandson left, and she continued with this routine. I tried various approaches, but I could see that being truthful with her was not working, so one day I told her, "Your Mom is on vacation in Italy," and I made up an elaborate story to go with this. That seemed to satisfy her for the time being. But of course, she would ask again, and I would have to repeat it. I asked her brother Tom and his family to go along with me in this, as it was the only thing that seemed to work.

One night, she was crying about her mother as she often did, and I told her, "Pretend I'm your mother." I proceeded to hold her and stroke her hair and cheeks as I imagined her mother would have done. This helped her a great deal, and she slept peacefully after that.

Bill hired someone to be with Maria while I was at work, but it didn't work out. Maria's family then decided, after a few daytime caregivers had come and gone, to take her to Atlanta for a month to stay with Joe and his family, and to get her tested for Alzheimer's. I would tell her that her son Joe was coming, but she had completely forgotten about him and even became angry: "I don't have a son named Joe!"

Joe's wife called me one night while Maria was at her brother Tom's house, and I explained the situation as best as I could. I said that I hoped they wouldn't institutionalize Maria. I felt that if she had a competent person in the daytime and the right medication, she would be fine. She promised that Maria would not be institutionalized. But the next time I talked to her, a month later, she said that Maria was coming home for a week and then was going into the Alzheimer's center nearby.

The week that Maria came home was one of the hardest times of my life. I cried most of the time, for I hated to see her go, and I also was in mourning for all we had meant to each other and for all the effort I had put in trying to help her.

I remembered the night awhile back when she was crying and saying she was afraid that they would come and take her away. I tried to reassure her, knowing that there was very little I could do.

The morning arrived. Bill called, saying that they were on their way. I hugged Maria and told her I loved her. I'll never forget her smiling face in the window as I backed out of the driveway on the way to work. How different it was now in January of 1989, a little over two years since I first saw her face in that very window.

As I write this, Maria has been in the center for over a year, and her condition has steadily worsened. It would no doubt have done so in any case.

What was this disease that destroyed Maria's life and had such an impact on the lives of those who were closest to her? What can caregivers do? And what about *our* spiritual and emotional needs? I'll try to give some answers in the following pages.

CHAPTER 2

Background Information

ALZHEIMER'S DISEASE, or AD, was first described by Alois Alzheimer in the early 1900s. Currently, Alzheimer's Disease is labeled Senile Dementia — Alzheimer's Type, abbreviated SDAT.

It had generally been believed that 2.5 million Americans were suffering from Alzheimer's. However, in a recent study, the National Institute on Aging concluded that the true figure is closer to 4 million. Although most Alzheimer's sufferers are over 65, some are younger.

Alzheimer's Disease is the fourth leading cause of death in this country, after heart disease, cancer, and stroke. It takes over 100,000 lives each year. Despite this, very few death certificates give Alzheimer's as the cause of death. Often, the victim is believed to have died from pneumonia. Actually, however, it is the brain's failure that causes death. The life expectancy of an Alzheimer's patient, when compared to the average elderly population, is reduced by up to one-third.

$123.4 million in federal funds was allocated to Alzheimer's research in 1989. In 1978, the figure was $5.1 million.

An estimated 10 to 30 percent of Alzheimer's patients have the type that is inherited. Roughly 70 percent of Alzheimer's sufferers remain at home, eventually needing round the clock attention. Families bear most of the burden of caring for these patients.

Alzheimer's could well be the most cruel of all diseases. It takes away one's dignity — not all at once, but gradually, in stages, so that the sufferer goes through a living hell. It causes a person to become as helpless as a child — and then as an infant — in mind and in body.

Alzheimer's Disease causes pathological changes in several areas of the brain, causing loss of mental ability, memory, and emotional control. Alzheimer's causes the brain's size and shape to alter. Because of the accelerated loss of brain cells, the brain shrinks and looks very old. The ventricles — inner spaces — of the brain increase in size, and the outer layer of cells becomes thinner and less dense.

It is part and parcel of Alzheimer's Disease that the symptoms vary from one patient to another, and that (as we saw in Maria's case) the symptoms change from day to day in the same patient. No single behavior or symptom is completely predictable, but the loss of recent memory seems to be universal.

This fact is among the most frustrating aspects of daily life with an Alzheimer's patient. A patient may talk what appears to be nonsense for days, and then have a lucid interval and talk quite normally. This is usually temporary, and soon the patient backslides. The pain of the victim and of his/her loved ones is enormous, as the family wonders how to treat their dear afflicted one. What makes him or her aware one moment, and disoriented and helpless at other times? Loss of memory is so painful, because we don't know who we are, or who our dear ones are. All that has happened in our lives — the good and the bad memories as well — are all erased, together with all that we have learned and striven for. We can't be sure we are loved, because our sense of security and reliability has turned into a very fragile web of uncertainty and fear. We become anxious and afraid, even of our dearest ones, on whom we depended all our lives.

Also, a person with Alzheimer's who is affected by some other disease, depression, fever or fatigue cannot recover as quickly. As the illness progresses, there is an unremittant physical and mental deterioration that usually occurs slowly over the years. However, at times, in some cases, it is a rapid and frightful progression.

Although there are variations with each person, there are four identifiable phases of Alzheimer's, each with its own peculiarities:

Phase One: The victim seems to have less energy, drive, and initiative. He or she is slower to react and learn new things. The Alzheimer's victim in this phase prefers to be around familiar people, places, and things. He or she avoids the unfamiliar, is less discriminating, and has catastrophic reactions, becoming easily upset and angered.

Phase Two: The patient's speech slows. One may not understand what is heard, lose the thread of a story, or miss the punchline of a simple joke. One may be unable to do simple arithmetic and need help with balancing a checkbook or doing other figuring. The person becomes increasingly self-absorbed, and seems totally insensitive to other people's feelings and needs. He or she avoids any situations that may end in failure. The individual in phase two is still able to function, but needs some supervision.

Phase Three: This phase is marked by obvious disability. The victim of Alzheimer's Disease is disoriented in regards to time and place, and cannot identify familiar people or events. This person can be very lethargic, invents his or her own words, and needs repeated instruction, encouragement, and direction. He or she may be most unsure of his or her self, behave in totally unexpected ways, and not express warmth as formerly to close friends and relatives. His or her memory of the distant past may be a vast improvement over recent memory, which is severely affected. This person's behavior changes considerably, and may take on bizarre and extreme forms.

Phase Four: This phase is, of course, the hardest of all to deal with. The patient is apathetic, and cannot find his or her way around the house or apartment in which he or she may have lived for several years. This person wanders, may be up during the night and ready to leave the house, and needs help with all the activities that are involved in daily life and self-care. He or she may have to be spoon-fed, or otherwise carefully supervised as to eating, drinking, as well as toilet and hygiene habits. The individual cannot tell whether things are hot or cold, and the disease also appears to affect the bodily thermostat, causing the victim to feel hotter or colder than would normally be the case.

Also in this phase, depression, delusions,

or delirium may occur. One loses many of one's inhibitions, and also may become incontinent.

Over the past 20 years, despite all the research that has thus far been done, no determination has yet been made as to why some people develop Alzheimer's Disease and others do not. However, Alzheimer's Disease does not respect one's intellectual capabilities, social or economic class, or occupation. Neither is there any answer at present as to what may cause Alzheimer's Disease, although unremitting stress, which lowers the effectiveness of the immune system, is thought to be a factor. Many different conditions, including nutritional deficiencies, chemical imbalances in the blood, tumors, and environmental stressors, such as metal poisoning from manganese or aluminum, may also lead to symptoms of recent memory loss. As yet, however, we do not know whether the accumulation of aluminum is a cause or an effect of Alzheimer's Disease.

A typical evaluation of a patient with suspected Alzheimer's Disease usually includes:

1) *a social and medical history.*
2) *a thorough physical examination.*
3) *a neuro-psychological examination.*
4) *sensory tests.*
5) *motor function.*
6) *face-hand test.*

7) *mental questionnaire.*
8) *memory for digits.*
9) *misplaced objects test.*
10) *paper and pencil tests.*
11) *PET SCAN.*
12) *EEG.*
13) *spinal tap.*
14) *blood tests.*
15) *brain biopsy (in very special cases).*

Potentially fruitful research continues, and we can only pray that effective treatments will be on the horizon. With our prayers and financial support of the Alzheimer's Disease and Related Disorders Association, this may be a reality someday soon.

In the meantime, the Alzheimer's patient needs constant care, attention, and emotional support from family and friends. Also, he or she needs protection and help as he or she becomes increasingly dependent.

What of the caregiver's needs? The following chapters will attempt to deal with these.

CHAPTER 3

Keeping Perspective

*Wanted: Caregiver for Alzheimer's patient.
Must be strong, loving, and wise. Must be
patient, and openminded. Must be responsive
24 hours a day. Must have a great deal of
patience and good health. Must be willing to
cope with any emergency, for little pay.*

THE ABOVE IS AN IMAGINARY AD, but it contains a
lot of truth in what is expected of the average
caregiver. An accumulation of events that happen to a caregiver over time can be most overwhelming. Most people are not prepared for
this. If I had been told that Maria had Alzheimer's before moving in with her, I wonder if I
really would have. But I do not regret my experiences. On the contrary, I feel that my life
has been enormously enriched because of having been with Maria.

Because Alzheimer's can take awhile before it progresses, that helps one to cope, in
some ways, and to adjust gradually. The

greatest thing to keep in mind is that you, the caregiver, have no doubt overcome previous challenges in your life, and you can draw on your own inner strengths to meet this challenge as well. You can acknowledge the illness, accepting the fact that, while the condition cannot be reversed (at least for the present), you can still care for the person, make him or her as comfortable as possible, and show kindness and affection. If you do not accept these things, your much needed resources will be drained out.

Take Life One Day at a Time. It is impossible to anticipate what might happen next in your patient's life, considering the seemingly infinite variables of this disease, mood swings, etc. Taking life one day at a time — even one hour at a time or less — is the most realistic thing you can do.

Your feelings, while trying to live this philosophy, will vary. You will feel fear of the unknown course ahead; sadness as you mourn a relationship that has changed drastically and will never be the same again; anger that you are going through this trial; despair when you feel you cannot cope; guilt when you worry that you haven't done everything you could for your patient, and for the times, in frustration, you vent your anger at the patient. You may also feel guilt because you may feel more anger than love under the daily stress of frustrations, and resentment when you no longer get your accustomed responses, or even so much as a "thank you." You will feel loneliness, an intense loneliness, because your life is no longer normal, because it is hard for you to keep up your social contacts as before, because you feel that nobody really understands, and, if they do, that they are too wrapped up in their own problems, because . . . the list goes on, and is as personal as the individuality of the caregiver.

Your feelings profoundly affect the way you deal with your patient, family members and friends, medical professionals, and others you come in touch with.

Whether you also have a spiritual life is important, and this cannot be emphasized enough. Maria was the kind of person who enjoyed going to Mass each Sunday. She had always been a religious person, and I know this helped her. Sometimes I would read the Bible to her, in Italian (because she could still remember Italian fairly well, and enjoyed hearing Scripture in the language of her youth) and in English, of course. I especially read the Beatitudes, the Psalms, and similar consoling passages of Scripture. This had a calming effect on both of us, and helped us face another day. Later on, I will touch more on the spiritual aspects of coping with this disease, keeping in mind that one's spiritual life is uniquely personal to each individual.

Support groups also help one to keep one's perspective. I was never able to attend one while I was with Maria, because the hours didn't coincide. However, my friends were my support group, and without them, I don't know how I could have gone on.

A patient who has been kind, loving, and gentle in his/her former life may be increasingly aggressive. Or one who has been an outgoing, take-charge type may be very simple, meek and childlike, asking permission for the least little thing. It is often difficult to keep one's patience through the countless situations that arise. Anger only serves to frustrate and confuse the patient more. You may have to ask yourself, when there is a disagreement or even a potential for one: Is this really worth it? Would this harm my patient if I didn't agree with him or her? What will this mean 10 years from now? If you both are alone watching the moon, for instance, and the patient says, "What a beautiful sun!", would it really be earth-shattering if you simply said "Yes, it's a beautiful sight, isn't it?" You will have to be an interpreter for your patient, who may have trouble finding the right words and will substitute whatever first comes to mind. Your patient may reach for the syrup container if he or she wants sugar in the coffee — Maria used to do this several times, and I said, "Here's your sugar," giving her the appropriate one, and hiding the syrup afterwards. If she told me or others in her family that she worked hard all day washing, ironing, and cleaning house, when we knew very well she didn't, we agreed with her to preserve her dignity. The patient is trying to salvage whatever dignity he or she has left — let us see to it that we help to preserve this dignity at all costs. Let us remember that, if life were arranged differently, *we* could have been the one with Alzheimer's, and our patient could have been *our* caregiver. How would we like to be treated? This also helps us to keep things in perspective. The Golden Rule, "Do unto others as you would have them do unto you," is certainly most useful in any situation, especially here.

You will feel angry, of course, but you will have to ventilate your anger in ways that your patient does not see. You may try cleaning closets, punching out pillows in your room, vigorous housecleaning or exercise, or, when possible, calling a trusted confidant. Ask for help! Don't feel that you must be a superman or superwoman! The caregiver is often called upon to do superhuman tasks, but we are all very human and very vulnerable. While we have to watch our emotional responses in front of our patient, we cannot bury our true selves inside. One of the most vulnerable times in my life was when I was with Maria, and I realized how very limited I was.

My major interests have always been music, art, and writing. I would often play records or tapes that I thought would be comforting both to Maria and myself. When we would travel in the car, we would sing . . . even when she couldn't remember all the words, she would make them up as she went along. She enjoyed it, and many tense moments were lightened up that way. We sometimes turned the radio off as we traveled and improvised our own versions of *76 Trombones* or a similarly rousing song, and laughed afterwards.

Laughter is also a wonderful thing to help keep things in perspective. We did a lot of that, especially when Maria was more lucid and could understand the humor in a situation and the punchlines of jokes. I was always looking for jokes to help lighten the atmosphere. Whereas we may at times have been frustrated with one another, the jokes helped us to grow closer.

Whatever talents you may have, I hope you will have the opportunities to utilize them. This will help to keep things in perspective. You are, after all, more than a caregiver. You are your own unique self, a very special individual made in God's image and likeness, with special talents, abilities, and aptitudes. You have your own history, your own personality, your own way of impacting on others, your own way of making this world a better place to live in because *you* are here. You must try to step outside of your caregiving role whenever possible to get your perspective. You cannot give what you do not have. You will feel guilty for arranging time off from your patient, especially when he or she shows displeasure, tears, or whatever. But you *must* take these times to get in touch with who you are, and your relationship to God and the world. You must let God fill you up again, to refresh and reinvigorate yourself.

If you are inclined to write, or even if you are not so inclined, writing also helps keep things in perspective. Write out your angry feelings in a letter to someone, then *throw it out!* It's amazing what a catharsis can happen by the very act of writing and getting your thoughts and feelings down on paper. Keep a journal, if possible, and lock it up afterwards. You may find encouragement by reading prior entries on how you survived various situations. You may find humor in certain situations that weren't so humorous at the time.

These are a few basic ideas, which may serve as a springboard for other ideas of your own. Keeping perspective is perhaps one of the most important things you can do for yourself *and* your patient!

CHAPTER 4

Listen To Your Feelings

"LISTEN TO *my* FEELINGS?" you may ask. "I have so many, I scarcely know where to begin!"

In Chapter 3, we have touched briefly on the feelings of: fear of the unknown, mourning of one's relationship with the Alzheimer's patient, anger, despair, guilt, frustration, and loneliness. In this chapter, we will now explore each of these feelings further.

Fear Of The Unknown. Most of us are afraid of the unknown, and we try to avoid it at all costs. Sometimes we succeed at it; sometimes not. We prefer that which is familiar and predictable. But the world of the Alzheimer's victim and his or her caregiver is anything *but* familiar and predictable. If a caregiver works outside the home, as I mentioned in my experience with Maria, he or she has no way of predicting what the home situation will be like tonight. Your patient may or may not be lucid and in a good mood; may have forgotten you were at work (or had to go out briefly for errands, as the case may be). Your patient may not recognize you. If there was another caregiver at home during the time of your absence, your patient may be angry at that caregiver and belligerent with you. The house may be in disorder; various things may have been moved somewhere they do not belong. If it is dark earlier, as in the case of fall and winter, your patient may already be in bed or preparing for bed.

Once you overcome whatever possible situation you find yourself in, and your patient has eaten and is safely tucked into bed for the night, there are more uncertainties, such as night wanderings. Your patient may arise at 3:00 A.M. and prepare to go out, or may bang the dresser drawers, or otherwise explore other areas of the house. Efforts to bring your patient back to bed may be successful at first, but very short-lived, as this may happen several times in the course of a night.

As you toss and turn at night, your fears become magnified as you think of the days, weeks, and months ahead. What will happen next? you wonder to yourself. How much longer will I be able to keep my sanity?

Mourning Of Your Relationship. Fear of the unknown course of the disease often leads to feelings of mourning for a relationship that you can no longer recover with your Alzheimer's patient, who may be a spouse, parent, brother or sister, or other close relative or friend. If the victim is your spouse, and you have relied on him or her to pay the bills, to keep the house running and in repair, to provide a sense of security and strength, to provide emotional and sexual support and intellectual companionship, you realize that none of this is possible anymore. Everything has drastically changed. If this patient is your Mom or Dad, and formerly provided you with maternal or paternal love and encouragement, a listening ear, guidance, and other forms of support, this is also gone. You are now a parent to your parent.

Anger. In your feelings of helplessness, fear and uncertainty, *anger* is the emotion that often comes next. You may be angry at God for allowing this to happen; angry at your patient for changing so; angry at others for not being supportive enough; angry at yourself for feeling angry!

Despair. Despair is a horrifying feeling, but one many caregivers pass through at one time or another. The thought that others have gone through it and have survived as stronger persons may be of comfort to you.

Guilt. This is probably one of the most frequent emotions a caregiver experiences. Some of them may have erroneously thought that if they were a better spouse, son, daughter, whatever, their spouse or parent would not have gone through this. Perhaps they should have encouraged their spouse or parent to read more, be more intellectually and socially active, get out of the house more, have less responsibilities and anxieties. But, you need to know that Alzheimer's is no respecter of persons in whatever intellectual, social, or financial status they may have enjoyed prior to the onset of the disease. You feel guilty when you get impatient or upset at your patient, and lash out in verbal abuse or in other displays of anger.

Frustration. You may find in the course of your day that you have answered the same question 20 times in ten minutes; finished washing the dishes and putting them away, only to be asked, "When are we going to eat?" You try to explain what seems to be a simple procedure over and over again, with no results. You do the 1001 tasks a caregiver does each day and night, knowing that the patient is never going to get better.

Loneliness. Spouses of an Alzheimer's patient have referred to themselves as "married widows" or "married widowers." Sex is often a turnoff. What communication exists is very brief and unsatisfying. You may try to treat your spouse as if he or she still understood, but you know that this is impossible. You cannot share comments even on TV programs, because TV is just a series of meaningless images to your patient. It is hard for you to leave your patient with someone trustworthy to socialize a bit; when you do, you still cannot stop worrying. People seldom come over or call because they feel awkward in the presence of this disease, which still carries a social stigma.

In the face of all this, how does one cope?

First of all, accept your feelings, whatever they may be. Don't compound them by feeling guilty for feeling guilty; angry for feeling angry, etc. These feelings need to be recognized and accepted for what they are, as normal reactions to an abnormal situation.

If you're feeling ill, you may need medical attention. If you are crying much of the time, not sleeping, unable to concentrate on anything, losing weight and having problems getting through the day, you may be suffering from a clinical depression that may require treatment, and should see a doctor or therapist.

If at all possible, ventilate your emotions to a trusted confidant, friend, priest, minister, rabbi, or medical or mental health person. Your patient is extremely sensitive to your feelings, regardless of the stage of the disease. Displays of anger or frustration worsen your tenuous relationship with your patient, who cannot understand your anger, and may become violent.

Because you cannot give what you do not have, if you wish to continue to maintain your physical and emotional health and well-being, and continue caring for your patient, you must do whatever is necessary to restore your equilibrium. Some suggestions are: attend a support group; use respite services (Call the local Alzheimer's chapter. If there is not one nearby, a local hospital or nursing home or mental health center may be able to assist you. Also, your pastor may be able to make referrals.) Exercise whenever possible. You may be quite exhausted indeed, but some moderate, pleasurable exercise has been shown to lift one's spirits. Try to get your patient to exercise with you — it will do you both a world of good. Take things in small, manageable steps. Try to acquire a sense of humor. Pray as much as you can, for God is with you!

CHAPTER 5

Spirituality And The Caregiver

ALONG WITH DEALING WITH YOUR EMOTIONS, and talking things out with a trusted confidant, your faith life is a very important consideration. Alzheimer's, like any other crisis in life, can cause one either to lose one's faith or to grow closer to God. In some cases, you may think that you have lost your faith — it may be merely dormant. With the many pressing cares you have to deal with, prayer, at least your former way of praying, may have fallen by the wayside. If this is the case, have hope, because what you are about to read may both surprise and encourage you!

You may have been taught a formal way of praying from missals, prayerbooks, and the like. You may thus have missed out on a lot of prayer, because you don't have either the time or the inclination to pray this way anymore — at least, not as often. In your depression and discouragement over your loved one's illness, you may feel that God is far from you, that He has perhaps abandoned you, that He has too many things on His mind running the universe to be concerned about you. Let us now consider your personal spirituality, and take each of these statements one at a time.

1) *I have always been taught to pray formally, and can no longer do so. How do I find the words to talk to God otherwise?*

There is no one method of prayer. There are times for formal prayer, but most often, prayer takes on very personal, private forms.

There is a story about a farmer who was unable to pray in the synagogue, because he had to till his fields. His Rabbi later asked him, "Tell me, when you were in the fields, did you pray?"

The farmer replied, "You know, Rabbi, I am not a learned man, and I do not know how to read. So when I was in the fields, I simply recited the alphabet, and asked God to form the letters into something that has meaning."

There is another story of a man who used to go to church every day after his work was done, and sit there and stare at the tabernacle. A priest noticed this, and finally approached the man, saying, "Every day I see you sitting here for hours, looking at the tabernacle. What do you find to say to Our Lord?"

The man replied, "Oh, I don't say much. I look at Him, He looks at me. We love each other. And when I leave, I feel happy."

Some people may say, "Good morning, God," and others may say, "Good God, morning!" These are also forms of prayer. Someone wrote: "I may be very busy today, God, and may forget Thee, but don't forget me!"

Many of us have known, at one time or another, at least one close personal friend that we felt comfortable enough with to talk to about anything on our minds, or even to keep silent for awhile, knowing that we were accepted and loved for who we are. Many beautiful and inspiring things have been written about the glories of friendship over the centuries. For example: "A friend is someone who knows all about you, and loves you just the same," or "A friend is someone who comes in when the whole world goes out."

God, of course, created the beautiful gift of friendship. He knows more about us than anyone, more than we ourselves, and loves us just the same. His love for us is unconditional. We don't have to prove ourselves to Him, or do great penances, or be unduly harsh with ourselves. We cannot buy His love, or earn it — it is always there. He has given us the free will to love Him in return if we so choose, and that is what He hopes for, but He will not force us to love Him. He shows His love through all His beautiful acts in creation, through countless ways.

But, when we suffer, we may feel tempted to say, "Well God, where's Your love now when I need it most? Have you abandoned me? Just look at this situation! Why do you permit so much suffering? Why do you permit my loved one to suffer from Alzheimer's, and my family and I as well?"

That, too, is prayer, being honest about our feelings, showing our anger at God. He is strong enough to take it. Besides, of what use would it be to try to hide anything from Him? Let us be completely ourselves with God, as we would be with a trusted friend, but even more so. All the friends of God, from the time of the Bible up to now, have been so open with God. We are no less important than they were. We need to remind ourselves of this, especially at times when, in our sufferings, our self-esteem suffers too.

2) *God seems so far away — how can I reach Him?*

There is a story about a man who went to a wise old sage and asked him how to find God. The sage smiled, said nothing, but led the man into a river where they waded as far as they could go. Then the sage forced the man's head under water. The man struggled violently for air, and, after a short while, the sage let him up again. As the man was choking and gasping, the sage asked him, "Tell me, when you were under water, what did you want most?"

"AIR!" the man gasped.

"When you seek God as much as you sought this air, you will find Him," the sage replied.

A little girl asked her mother how to find God. The mother told her child to place her hand on her pulse, and as she did so, said, "Whenever you need to feel that God is present with you, just feel your pulse, because He is as close as that."

Yes, God is in our pulse, He is as close as the very air we breathe. If we take a moment to breathe in slowly and deliberately, and imagine that God is filling our very beings (although He is already there inside of us), we realize that He is the one who has created us and sustains us in life. It is impossible for Him to forget us, for, if He did so, we would surely vanish. As we breathe out, let us feel that His love and care extends to all around us, all whom we love (especially, in this case, our Alzheimer's victim), and all our concerns.

Our God is an ever present refuge in time

of trouble, yearning to help us if we only turn to
Him. We may feel the full brunt of our weakness and powerlessness — especially in the face
of Alzheimer's Disease, as we watch the deterioration of our patient, knowing that there is very
little that we can do, other than to try to make
him or her as comfortable as possible. God's
strength is made perfect in our weakness.
Would we turn to Him if everything went our
way all the time? Probably not. It is in those
times that He is most often forgotten. Let us try
to make a habit of practicing the presence of
God in our good times, whenever they may
come, so that it will be easier to continue in our
hard times as well.

3) *Sometimes God seems like a busy executive running the universe. With so
many things to remember, it is hard
for me to think He would be concerned with me and the details of my
life.*

Reflect for a moment that every snowflake,
every leaf, every stone is different. Yet
these things seem inconsequential to us — what
does it really matter? Think that if God cared
enough to worry about the details of these
small, minute things, how much more does He
care for us living, breathing, human beings!
Well, we ask, why aren't my prayers answered?

Why is there so much suffering and so little variety in my life? A million whys. . . .

Trying to know these answers with any certainty is like trying to stuff the ocean into a seashell! But one thing we do know is this: we are co-creators with God. We have been given unique sets of personalities, strengths, and weaknesses that no other person has. All of us have been created to love God in a way that no one else can, and to make our contribution to the world in whatever way we can, however small and insignificant it seems.

Suppose all the inventors thought to themselves, before making their inventions (or halfway finished with them), "Well, this is just a crazy idea! People will laugh at me, and it just doesn't seem so important after all." We would probably still be living in caves! Fortunately for us, they persevered until what they had was something workable, and this something, whether it was the invention of the wheel or of electric lights, had an almost limitless impact in our world for generations!

Someone wrote, "Please be patient, God isn't finished with me yet!" We are still being created, still being made anew, whatever contrary evidence may appear at the present time. We have only to think how we have grown and changed over the years. The people we have known, the relationships we have entered into, everything that has either happened to us or we have caused to happen, has had an impact on our lives and the lives of others. No, God is not a busy executive running the universe, too busy to care about the details of our lives. He is very much involved, more than we can ever imagine!

The following poem shows what a difference it can make in our lives, when we try to practice the awareness of God's presence and turn to Him. It is called, appropriately enough, *The Difference:*

The Difference

I got up early one morning
and rushed right into the day;
I had so much to accomplish
that I didn't have time to pray.
Problems just tumbled about me,
and heavier came each task,
"Why doesn't God help me?" I wondered.
He answered, "You didn't ask."
I wanted to see joy and beauty,
but the day toiled on, gray and bleak,
I wondered why God didn't show me.
He said, "But you didn't seek."
I tried to come into God's presence;
I used all my keys at the lock.
God gently and lovingly chided,

"My child, you didn't knock."
I woke up early this morning,
and paused before entering the day;
I had so much to accomplish
that I had to take time to pray.

CHAPTER 6

Psychotherapy And Pastoral Care

ASKING FOR HELP IS HARD TO DO, especially in our American culture, where so much emphasis is placed on self-sufficiency and independence. But sooner or later, we come face to face with the facts: namely, that we are *not* self-sufficient or independent. We are sufficient only to a certain extent, and we are *interdependent*. As we have discussed in Chapter 5, we literally depend on God to keep us in existence. He has also made us social beings. In Chapter 5, we have also dealt with some qualities of friendship.

At times of crisis, family or friends are usually turned to first for support, and this is often quite successful. But where this is not, if someone is able to afford it, one goes for psychotherapy. Pastoral care is also another very viable option.

I have chosen to discuss psychotherapy

and pastoral care in this chapter because they have many similarities. First, let's look at psychotherapy:

Individual psychotherapy can be very useful for anyone whose internal conflicts prevent him or her from participating more fully in life. It helps to alleviate fears and worries that may be hindrances to personal and career successes. Especially in the case of one who is a caregiver for an Alzheimer's patient, psychotherapy offers relief from the feeling of "going it alone," and from the emotions that run rampant in such a situation. A skilled psychotherapist can often help one to uncover underlying conflicts, work through anxiety-producing situations and the concomitant negative feelings that arise, and find creative options to dealing with internal stress and stressful life situations.

In group psychotherapy, family members who share the problems of living with an Alzheimer's victim can learn how to get along better with each other, and how to improve their relationship with their memory-impaired patient. They learn to understand their feelings of anger, guilt, resentment, frustration and anxiety, and develop ways of dealing with these feelings. Practical skills and ways of managing the Alzheimer's patient at home are also dealt with, as well as discussions about the future and the possibilities of having to institutionalize the Alzheimer's patient. Also in group therapy, caregivers can develop a more accepting attitude toward their patient and themselves. It lessens the feeling of isolation one experiences, and provides the feeling of being really understood by others who are co-sufferers.

Likewise, in pastoral care, opportunities are also provided for individual counseling and group therapy in certain parishes, Catholic hospitals, etc. While there are some differences in training and the obvious difference of cost factors, those in pastoral care are able to offer the very important spiritual perspective and dimension to coping with Alzheimer's Disease. While this sometimes happens in psychotherapy, it is generally more the exception than the norm.

But whether you choose individual or group psychotherapy or pastoral care, the following considerations are very important and can help you derive the most benefit from your sessions:

If you can feel that your therapy is a joint exploration embarked upon by you and your therapist, it will be quite valuable to you. By reviewing your life and the losses you have experienced, you will be enabled to express how you feel about these losses, and what they mean to you. You will be able to replace painful attitudes and behaviors with new, more positive ones. By sharing your anger and other painful feelings with your therapist, you will be enabled to think and feel more positive.

An empathetic therapist will understand how you feel, and provide a safe haven in which to deal with corrective experiences and risk-taking. The confidentiality of your sessions will enable you to feel more free to discuss things that would otherwise make you feel ashamed or embarrassed to bring out into the open.

Like all relationships, it takes time to develop trust and confidence in your therapist or pastoral care counselor. There may be things about the therapist or therapy that displease you, or with which you may feel uncomfortable. It is important to be open about these things also, and not to let yourself be too intimidated by your therapist or counselor.

Most qualified therapists or pastoral care workers do not continue the relationship longer than needed. If you are considering psychotherapy and are looking for a qualified therapist, check a local or national directory to see that the therapist in question has the appropriate education and credentials. Two directories you may want to look into are those of the American Psychological Association and the National Association for the Advancement of Psychoanalysis. On your first visit, you should discuss credentials, fee, length and frequency of sessions, and the confidentiality issue.

When looking into pastoral care, it is also a certainty that academic credentials and/or expertise will differ. However, it is also true that, as with any profession or occupation, some are more naturally gifted than others, and this should also be taken into consideration. You may ask yourself what your expectations are. No one person may be able to meet them all. But between a network of family, friends, and your choice of either or both psychotherapy and pastoral care, your chances of maintaining your overall health will be that much stronger, as well as your ability to keep your memory-impaired loved one home longer. Since it has been found that the psychological and otherwise general health of caregivers deteriorates more rapidly the longer the caregiving role is continued, the emphasis on supportive measures cannot be too strong.

Knowing that you have done your level best to cope as long as possible with the effects of the disease on your memory-impaired loved one will greatly serve to lessen the overwhelming feelings of guilt and depression which often accompany placement in a nursing home, or upon the death of the Alzheimer's victim — whichever comes first.

Also, the self-knowledge you will have gained through whatever therapeutic avenue you chose will be of inestimable value. You have done much good for your Alzheimer's patient. Your patient, whether directly or indirectly, will also have ministered to you in helping you to see life in a whole new light, in helping you to know yourself better, as well as learning more about the giftedness you have in certain areas, and the potentials of which you are capable. In recent years, more and more books on the subject of Wounded Healers have appeared. You, as well as your Alzheimer's victim, each in your own ways, have truly become Wounded Healers, the significance of which may never be fully known in this life, but surely in the next.

CHAPTER 7

Practical Tips

SOMETHING ELSE that cannot be emphasized enough is the importance of organization in caring for your Alzheimer's patient. The following tips are meant to be a general guide — you may also have other ideas which would be helpful for you and your patient in living a more peaceful, structured life (or at least as much of a structured life as you can have under the circumstances.)

1) As much as possible, keep to a routine, which will lessen the aggravation and confusion for your patient, who finds it hard to adapt to even the most simple duties we take for granted every day, such as cleaning, washing, dressing, eating, etc.

2) Consistent behavior is crucial. Your patient suffers from rapidly changing moods, as well as his or her struggles with doing tasks such as eating, sleeping, taking a bath, taking medication, or whatever. He or she may overreact to your requests by swearing, sobbing, or with

physical or verbal abuse. Be very softspoken, and break everything down into very simple, manageable steps — and, as has been mentioned before, control your anger and frustration, which would only escalate your problems. Don't try to argue or to reason with your patient. Take some deep breaths and try to keep calm, take your loved one's hand gently and speak softly. Afterwards, vent your anger and frustration by talking them out with a friend, or by doing some housework, exercise, or anything else that would be practical and useful.

3) Consider everything in your home — how is it set up? Are electric appliances, like irons, hair dryers, sewing machines, saws and drills locked up? Are medicine, household cleaners, and other dangerous items out of sight and out of reach? Are exposed pipes concealed? What about access to the hot water heater and furnace?

Are extension cords and slippery rugs tacked down?

Are fragile knick-knacks and valuable items put away?

Bright lighting is needed, as well as conveniently placed handrails, and stairs with reflector treads and a gate at the top. Support bars may be needed in bathrooms, as well as a slip-proof mat in the tub, and good overflow drains in the tub and sink, so that if your patient leaves the water running, there will be no flood.

In the kitchen, knives and other dangerous implements should be out of sight and reach. The knobs should be removed from the stove.

Locks on exterior doors should be placed at the top or bottom, out of reach of the impaired person, and perhaps disguised in such a way that they cannot be easily recognized and tampered with.

Also, it is very important to keep the tension levels down in the house as much as possible, because there is a direct correlation between rising tension and increased accidents in the home.

In the bedroom, it is helpful to put the Alzheimer's patient's bed next to the wall, so that he or she could only get out on one side and avoid confusion.

Somewhere in the house, there should be a wall calendar, a wall clock, and a chart of activities that could be checked off together with your patient after he or she performs little chores like watering the plants, making the beds, etc. This could help your patient to feel more useful. Also, a little sign could be placed nearby giving today's date, time, and perhaps even weather conditions, thus helping your patient be oriented to reality.

Labels, pictures, and notes on things

around the house also help your patient to maintain more confidence and independence. Put labels on all the drawers, broom closet, bathroom, etc., with perhaps pictures or drawings of the contents.

Tell your friends and acquaintances when you'll be available to speak with them by phone, or that you'll call them. This will help eliminate problems with the telephone, because your confused loved one can no longer handle messages and may actually tell the person calling that you're out when you're standing right there. An answering machine hidden somewhere in the house can also be helpful in this regard.

Provide a bracelet that has your loved one's name, address, telephone number, and the words "Memory Impaired" on it. This would save a lot of grief in the event your patient wanders off. Most hospital gift shops sell ID bracelets such as these. They are also available from Medic Alert. The Medic Alert ID is made of metal, and can be worn as a necklace or bracelet, on the back of which is engraved the patient's ID number and medical condition, along with a 24-hour telephone number. In a central file at that number, available to whoever makes a collect call, is vital information such as the patient's name, address, telephone number, nearest relative, and the family doctor's name, address, and telephone number. The Medic Alert Foundation International, which is located at Turlock, California 95380, telephone 209-632-2371 is a charitable organization that charges a one-time-only membership fee.

Since each patient is different, each caregiver will have opportunities to be creative in dealing with whatever needs arise. But the above-mentioned suggestions are helpful in most cases. With the advancement of the disease, however, even the most well-meaning of efforts can fail. Caregivers will sooner or later be forced to ask themselves what would be best for all concerned. If a caregiver cannot cope, with or without outside help, a serious examination of matters must be done, and eventually nursing homes may be taken into consideration.

... medical examinations and reimbursement ... The Atomic Alert Radiation Instrument, Model E-520 (reprice @ $157.2). It is challenging ... organizations that choose ... inexpensively to medical staff ...

Since each person is duty-free, firms are given full responsibilities to be creative in dealing with whatever goods enter the purchase inventory. Suggestions are half out in most cases. With the advantage of the discussion, however, here the most well-thought-of efforts on the part. Enterprises will support in any necessary forced to set the goods they have would be best for all concerned. If presented, a major problem with or without remedy helps to escape complaints. If major demand must become another, an existing problem may be taken into consideration.

CHAPTER 8

Nursing Homes

WHEN NURSING HOMES come to mind, many emotions, thoughts and feelings rise to the surface. Most people tend to think of nursing homes with disgust and aversion. For many, the thought of living in a nursing home is associated with feelings of uselessness, loneliness, and abandonment. Fearing that a loved one may be mistreated in such a place drives many families to go to extreme measures to keep their Alzheimer's victim at home — in his or her own home, if possible, or in the home of an adult child or nearest relative.

The decision to place one's dear Alzheimer's patient in a nursing home is quite difficult, and gives rise to much emotion. One of the first emotions is guilt, especially in families where the 4th commandment of "Honor thy father and thy mother" has often been emphasized strongly. One may be facing feelings of anger at the Alzheimer's victim for having to be placed in this situation, and at oneself for feelings of failure and inadequacy at having tried to deal with all the ramifications of this terrible disease. Also, there is anger among family members, each pointing an accusing finger at the other, even at the one who was good enough to try to be principal caregiver. The caregiver, in turn, may be angry at the perceived lack of support from family members, or insufficient support, whether real or imagined. These intense feelings of anger, unless appropriately dealt with, admitted to, talked out, etc., could be turned inward and result in depression.

Over the past several years, I have been in nursing homes in different states, and I have seen a variety of environments and of treatments received by the patients.

I have seen nursing homes in which patients are restrained in chairs all day long, sometimes sitting in their own waste, fed small portions of unpalatable foods, are overly medicated, and, in general, treated most impersonally, coldly and uncaringly, by the staff. And I have seen nursing homes where quite the opposite is true: where the staff sincerely tries to care for the overall well-being of each patient entrusted to their care.

In addition, nursing home scandals that have been reported in the media over the last ten years or so have sometimes given the public a negative image of nursing homes, much like the image of the "snake pit" for the mentally disturbed of former times.

However, current nursing home abuses have been reduced or largely eliminated. Each state has strict regulations by which nursing homes must abide, and inspections are made regularly. There is a Patient's Bill of Rights, and nursing homes are subject to severe penalties if the rights of a resident are violated.

Depending on the uniqueness of each individual, some may adjust well to nursing homes; others may rapidly deteriorate, despite the efforts of the most well-meaning staff and family members and friends. It is very important to know this and to be accepting of this fact in either case.

Nursing homes have their particular ways of determining the care level needed by a resident. The level-of-care rating establishes what services are necessary for a patient's care, and a board periodically reviews all nursing home patients. Alzheimer's patients, because of their special needs, are not accepted into just any nursing home. There are some which specialize in this care, and this number will probably grow as the need increases. Also, the level-of-care rating can also determine Medicare and Medicaid eligibility, and payment level. An evaluation form to obtain this level-of-care rating will need to be filled out by your doctor after a recent medical examination.

How can you evaluate a nursing home? There are questions which you should ask, and answers you have a right to know. You should be able to inspect the facilities and find out about the types of medical and nursing services which are available, and investigate these services, the administration and staff. If they do not allow you to do this, or hinder you from speaking to the residents, or hedge about an exact itemization of costs in a certain nursing home, forget that place and go elsewhere. Try to answer your own questions through your own observation, if possible, but if you are in doubt, ask the administration and/or members of the staff.

Objective ratings about nursing homes may be obtained from The Long-Term Care Council of the Joint Commission on Accreditation of Hospitals, or The American Health Care Association. Other licensing approvals you should look for are memberships in a State Nursing Home Association, American Association of Homes for the Aging, and/or the American Nursing Home Association, as well as a Nursing Home Administration license.

Licensing by the proper state authorities should be openly displayed. The licensing codes prescribe requirements for fire safety, nutrition, type of staff, and the number of people necessary to attend to patients and their needs.

Three very important areas to discuss with nursing home administration are: accreditation, financial procedures, and quality of residential care. The only one you can generally obtain in writing is a copy of the financial arrangements, which specify costs that are basically included in the charge, and those which are extra. Sometimes there are additional charges for medications, special nursing procedures, incontinence pads, laundry, beauty parlor, and aides to help your patient to exercise. Make sure also that the home is certified to accept Medicare or Medicaid, and also that the home will continue to keep a privately-paying patient who is switched to Medicaid.

An Alzheimer's facility should encourage a family to bring some of the patient's personal items to make him or her feel more at home.

Check to see if there are regular fire drills, and if the safety requirements such as good lighting, grab bars, handrails, etc. are being followed.

Consider food services, and see if there is a licensed dietician in charge of the kitchen. Ask if special diets can be obtained, if between meal and bedtime snacks are available, and whether patients are fed if they cannot eat by themselves. How soon are trays removed after eating?

You will, of course, also be interested in the condition of patients' rooms, to see if they are cheerful, well lit, and not too crowded.

You will also want to see the dining and recreation areas, visiting areas, etc. and see if they are well-attended.

Some homes provide calendars of events which list all the social activities for each day. An Alzheimer's Center of which I am familiar does this on a regular basis, and it is refreshing to see the wide variety of activities which are available for anyone wanting to make use of them. However, it should also be remembered that one who has not been used to too much activity, and prefers a quieter life with a few visitors, TV and radio should be respected.

It is well, if possible, to enlist the services of a professional social worker, psychologist, or professionally trained gerontologist in helping a caregiver and family's decisions about placing their loved one in a home, and, upon placement, to help the patient and family cope with this traumatic new phase of their lives.

It should be remembered that placement of a loved one in a nursing home will be far from easy, even if it has been done relatively peacefully and successfully. The feelings of doubt, despair, or ambivalence that have occurred previously will return in somewhat different ways, perhaps, and be accompanied by several other feelings, such as loneliness and emptiness, especially for the caregiver, whose every moment had been filled to the brim attending to the patient.

It is important to accept these feelings as normal, to realize that there is nothing wrong with you. There is a grief period which must follow, as you grieve over what has been lost: the loss of your loved one's memory, and all that goes along with that; the loss of your former relationship, which will never be the same again, at least on this earth; the loss of all the time you spent, all the emotional, spiritual, physical, as well as financial energy that went into caring for your Alzheimer's patient, knowing that all you have done could not halt the progress of the disease or cure your patient; the loss of all you used to be, of all your feelings and thoughts about how life should be and should have been.

Also, the decline of a once powerful parent or spouse is most painful, and makes us aware that we too will one day die. We must face the fact that we will age, and perhaps suffer a similar fate. The thought that death is inevitable, both for our loved ones and ourselves, is too much to bear. We may prefer to block out these feelings and thoughts, but we need to confront them with a supportive friend, pastoral care worker, or other experienced counselor or psychotherapist. Thus we will find strength, and we will realize that, no matter what we may think to the contrary, God does not give us more than we can bear, but gives us the grace to come to terms with any situation and to rise above it. Even after the worst of winters, there is a beautiful spring; after the darkest night, there is the light of day. Each year we celebrate Easter. We try to comprehend its meaning, that Christ rose victoriously, and we will too, and all tears will be wiped from our eyes. It is hard to comprehend this, but we need to believe that we will one day experience the reality of Easter. We need to be convinced that God, Who brought us thus far, will be faithful and take us all the way to Him, and that there *really* is a reason for everything, even, and especially in this case, Alzheimer's Disease, and its effects on our lives. Indeed, it has often been said that watching an Alzheimer's patient suffer throughout all the stages of the disease is like being at an endless funeral. But because of our Christian faith, we believe in God and that He offers us eternal life! The concept of eternal life, filled with love, joy, happiness and peace, is really mind-boggling when you just consider the word *eternal* as literally meaning without end.

St. Paul wrote in Ephesians 1:18-20, "I ask that your minds be open to see his light, so that you will know what is the hope to which he has called you, how rich are the wonderful blessings he promises his people, and how very great is his power at work in us who believe. This power working in us is the same as the mighty strength which he used when he raised Christ from death and seated him at his right side in the heavenly world." (Good News Version)

May we nourish ourselves with Scripture, and find much strength and encouragement therein! In the meantime, let us say the words of Psalm 62:

> I wait patiently for God to save me;
>   I depend on him alone.
> He alone protects and saves me; he is my
>   defender, and I shall never be de-
>   feated.
> Trust in God at all times, my people.
> Tell him all your troubles,
>   for he is our refuge.   (vs. 1-2, 8)

CHAPTER 9

A Word To Pastors

SO FAR, this little book has been addressed mainly to caregivers of Alzheimer's patients. In the last chapter, I briefly mentioned some of the reasons that a caregiver should seek pastoral counseling.

The focus in this chapter is a bit different. It's addressed to the pastor or other minister who might be faced with trying to help a caregiver and his or her patient.

Many churches and dioceses now hold support group meetings for Alzheimer's caregivers and their families. However, a large number of caregivers are unable or unwilling to attend such meetings.

Firstly, the great demands made on the time and attention of caregivers may make it difficult or impossible for them to attend such meetings.

Secondly, the caregiver is very vulnerable. It often happens that the caregiver's family and friends are not very supportive. This loneliness and stress often cause the caregiver to feel alienated from God, church, and prayer. A question frequently in the caregiver's heart is: "Why did God allow my dear one to get Alzheimer's? What did he (or she) ever do to deserve this? What did I ever do?" The caregiver needs to know that his/her church or synagogue is concerned for both caregiver and patient.

Thirdly, caregivers may not approach pastors or pastoral ministers because of the stigma attached to senility in our society. Caregivers are very much aware of this stigma, and frequently use every means at their disposal to keep up appearances.

Ironically, this struggle to keep up appearances often creates problems with the caregiver's family and friends — not to mention the patient's family! It's amazing how long a clean and well-groomed Alzheimer's patient can maintain his or her social graces, even when the disease has been advancing for some time. People may say, "Well, Jim (or Mary) looks fine to me. I don't know what all the fuss is about!" In fact, that very morning, Jim might have gotten lost in his own house, or Mary might have been crying because her long-dead father never came around to see her any more.

Here are a few suggestions on ministering to Alzheimer's patients and caregivers:

Alzheimer's Disease could be mentioned in the Prayers of the Faithful. For example, "For victims of Alzheimer's Disease and their caregivers and loved ones, that they may know the healing touch of Jesus, we pray to the Lord."

Unofficial healing services for Alzheimer's patients and caregivers could be held. The book *Pastoral Care of the Sick*, published by the Catholic Book Publishing Company of New York, is a rich source for ideas for such services.

Alzheimer's could be mentioned in homilies. A sample homily will be found in the next chapter.

Pamphlets on Alzheimer's could be displayed in racks. See the resource listing at the end of this book for where to get such pamphlets.

How about your homebound parishioners? Some of them may have Alzheimer's or a related disorder.

How many people are going around with this disease — yet in the early stages, perhaps, — who are afraid to be tested because they feel they cannot cope, or because they might not have the necessary insurance? Certain cases of depression, too much medication, brain tumors, or other diseases can mimic Alzheimer's. People need to be educated about these things.

Or how many people in the early stages of Alzheimer's Disease fear that they are losing their minds and are candidates for insane asylums? They could find comfort in knowing that they have a disease which can be treated, up to a point.

How many caregivers — often close family members — are living with the overwhelming fear that the disease is hereditary in their family, and that they might be the next victim?

Some of your parishioners may not be listed as homebound. They may simply have discontinued church attendance. This, of course, is caused by a variety of factors. But *some* of this group may be afflicted with Alzheimer's. They, like all the rest, need reaching out to.

Then again, some caregivers may approach you or your staff. It may be in sheer desperation — they see the beginning signs of Alzheimer's and don't know where to turn. Or they may have read or heard some recent mention of Alzheimer's Disease in a parish bulletin, a pamphlet, a newspaper notice, prayer, or a homily. In such cases, the information I have given in Chapter 5 on the spiritual and psychological needs of caregivers may be of assistance to you.

In the facility where Maria lives, one of the Alzheimer's patients is a priest. It can strike anyone, anywhere, at any time. Pastors and religious superiors need to be aware of this, and have some type of preparations ready. As often happens, we don't fully appreciate a problem unless it somehow impacts on us directly. Thus, your awareness of this may well be useful for you or someone you know sometime in the future.

CHAPTER 10

A Sample Homily

"I AM WITH YOU." Jesus said these words on many occasions. He displayed them in His actions. "I am with you." These words have power. They are a comfort to us when we need to hear them the most, when we are in desperate situations and feel vulnerable and alone. Many of us here today are burdened down with great hardships and loneliness. We here at _____ parish are deeply concerned about each of you, and are here to listen and help you in any way we can.

Today, I wish to address those of you who are caregivers for Alzheimer's victims, those of you who are friends of such caregivers, and those of you who suspect that a friend or relative may have Alzheimer's Disease.

This tragic disease affects some 4 million Americans, and is our country's fourth largest killer, after heart disease, cancer and stroke. Although it mostly affects people over 65, many victims are much younger. It attacks the brain, affecting first the memory and emotions, and later on, bodily functions.

As we get older, most of us experience some normal memory loss. But when such memory loss begins to affect our daily activities, something is seriously wrong. It may not necessarily be Alzheimer's Disease. There are other disorders that affect the memory, and some of these can be treated and cured. As yet, however, there is no known cure for Alzheimer's Disease. Research for such a cure is being done around the clock. November is National Alzheimer's Disease Awareness Month. I encourage everyone who possibly can, to learn more about Alzheimer's Disease and to donate to local or national chapters of the Alzheimer's Disease and Related Disorders Association.

You caregivers of Alzheimer's victims should be commended for your heroic efforts in trying daily to comfort the suffering. You are suffering victims also, though in a different way. You see through your loving eyes how Alzheimer's Disease can turn a loved one into a stranger, how it can strip away memory, intelligence and personality. You truly put the love of Christ into action. Like Jesus, you too can say, "I am with you." The Alzheimer's Association has a similar motto: "Someone to stand by you." You are not alone, humanly or divinely.

"Do not reject me now that I am old; do not

abandon me now that I am feeble." These words could be spoken by an Alzheimer's victim. They are from Psalm 71. Further on, the same Psalm reads, "Now that I am old and my hair is gray, do not abandon me, O God! . . . You have sent troubles and suffering on me, but you will restore my strength. . . . You will make me greater than ever; you will comfort me again."

Love, however, is something that endures — if not in words, then in feelings and gestures. Love is the sign we can give to our Alzheimer's patient, to show that he or she has not been abandoned or rejected by us or by God. A hug, a gentle handclasp, a smile, a warm glance — these communicate love more eloquently than words can.

You know how much your Alzheimer's patient needs these loving gestures more than ever before. He or she is trying to cope with a world that is crumbling into pieces. Through the eyes of Alzheimer's, everything is seen differently.

Let us never lose hope or prayer in the midst of these trials and hardships. It may seem that God is far away, but He is not. In Christ, He says, "I am with you always." He keeps His promises.

Let us hold fast to Christ as our strong Anchor in the storm, and let us pray without ceasing that a cure for Alzheimer's may soon be found. Meanwhile, let us also pray for one another, for the strong love and faith we need to carry our daily burdens, whatever they may be, until the day when we shall meet in heaven and, as our Lord says, "every tear shall be wiped from your eyes." The eyes of Alzheimer's will one day be victorious eyes, strong, loving, and happy. On that day, we will learn why all this had to be.

May God richly bless you.   Amen.

CHAPTER 11

Scripture Readings

Psalm 71:9-21

Do not cast me off in the time of old age;
forsake me not when my strength is spent. For
my enemies speak concerning me, those who
watch for my life consult together, and say,
"God has forsaken him; pursue and seize him,
for there is none to deliver him." O God, be not
far from me; O my God, make haste to help me!
May my accusers be put to shame and con-
sumed; with scorn and disgrace may they be
covered who seek my hurt. But I will hope
continually, and will praise thee yet more and
more. My mouth will tell of thy righteous acts,
of thy deeds of salvation all the day, for their
number is past my knowledge. With the mighty
deeds of the Lord God I will come, I will praise
thy righteousness, thine alone. O God, from my
youth thou hast taught me, and I still proclaim
thy wondrous deeds. So even to old age and
gray hairs, O God, do not forsake me, till I
proclaim thy might to all the generations to

come. Thy power and thy righteousness, O God, reach the high heavens. Thou who hast done great things, O God, who is like thee? Thou who hast made me see many sore troubles wilt revive me again; from the depths of the earth thou wilt bring me up again. Thou wilt increase my honor, and comfort me again.

Psalm 143:1-8
Hear my prayer, O Lord; give ear to my supplications! In thy faithfulness answer me, in thy righteousness! Enter not into judgment with thy servant; for no man living is righteous before thee. For the enemy has pursued me; he has crushed my life to the ground; he has made me sit in darkness like those long dead. Therefore my spirit faints within me; my heart within me is appalled. I remember the days of old, I meditate on all thou hast done; I muse on what thy hands have wrought. I stretch out my hands to thee; my soul thirsts for thee like a parched land. Make haste to answer me, O Lord! My spirit fails! Hide not thy face from me, lest I be like those who go down to the Pit. Let me hear in the morning of thy steadfast love, for in thee I put my trust. Teach me the way I should go, for to thee I lift up my soul.

Isaiah 43:1-7
But now thus says the Lord, he who created

you, O Jacob, he who formed you, O Israel: "Fear not, for I have redeemed you; I have called you by name, you are mine. When you pass through the waters I will be with you; and through the rivers, they shall not overwhelm you; when you walk through fire you shall not be burned, and the flame shall not consume you. For I am the Lord your God, the Holy One of Israel, your Savior. I give Egypt as your ransom, Ethiopia and Seba in exchange for you. Because you are precious in my eyes, and honored, and I love you, I give men in return for you, peoples in exchange for your life. Fear not, for I am with you; I will bring your offspring from the east, and from the west I will gather you; I will say to the north, Give up, and to the south, Do not withhold; bring my sons from afar and my daughters from the end of the earth, every one who is called by my name, whom I created for my glory, whom I formed and made."

Sirach 3:10-16
Do not glorify yourself by dishonoring your father, for your father's dishonor is no glory to you. For a man's glory comes from honoring his father, and it is a disgrace for children not to respect their mother. O son, help your father in his old age, and do not grieve him as long as he lives; even if he is lacking in understanding,

show forbearance; in all your strength do not despise him. For kindness to a father will not be forgotten, and against your sins it will be credited to you; in the day of your affliction it will be remembered in your favor; as frost in fair weather, your sins will melt away. Whoever forsakes his father is like a blasphemer, and whoever angers his mother is cursed by the Lord.

Matthew 5:3-10
Blessed are the poor in spirit, for theirs is the kingdom of heaven.

Blessed are those who mourn, for they shall be comforted.

Blessed are the meek, for they shall inherit the earth.

Blessed are those who hunger and thirst after righteousness, for they shall be satisfied.

Blessed are the merciful, for they shall obtain mercy.

Blessed are the pure in heart, for they shall see God.

Blessed are the peacemakers, for they shall be called sons of God.

Blessed are those who are persecuted for righteousness' sake, for theirs is the kingdom of heaven.

Romans 8:26-27, 31-32, 35, 37-39

Likewise the Spirit helps us in our weakness; for we do not know how to pray as we ought, but the Spirit himself intercedes for us with sighs too deep for words. And he who searches the hearts of men knows what is the mind of the Spirit, because the Spirit intercedes for the saints according to the will of God. . . . What then shall we say to this? If God is for us, who is against us? He who did not spare his own Son but gave him up for us all, will he not also give us all things with him? . . . Who shall separate us from the love of Christ? Shall tribulation, or distress, or persecution, or famine, or nakedness, or peril, or the sword? . . . No, in all these things we are more than conquerors through him who loved us. For I am sure that neither death, nor life, nor angels, nor principalities, nor things present, nor things to come, nor powers, nor heights, nor death, nor anything else in all creation will be able to separate us from the love of God in Christ Jesus our Lord.

2 Corinthians 4:7-12, 16-18; 5:1

But we have this treasure in earthen vessels, to show that the transcendent power belongs to God and not to us. We are afflicted in every way, but not crushed; perplexed, but not driven to despair; persecuted, but not forsaken; struck down, but not destroyed; always carrying in the body the death of Jesus, so that the life of Jesus may also be manifested in our bodies. For while we live we are always being given up to death for Jesus' sake, so that the life of Jesus may be manifested in our mortal flesh. So death is at work in us, but life in you. . . . So we do not lose heart. Though our outer nature is wasting away, our inner nature is being renewed every day. For this slight momentary affliction is preparing for us an eternal weight of glory beyond all comparison, because we look not to the things that are seen but to the things that are unseen; for the things that are seen are transient, but the things that are unseen are eternal. For we know that if the earthly tent we live in is destroyed, we have a building from God, a house not made with hands, eternal in the heavens.

Suggested Readings

Alzheimer's Disease: A Guide for Families. Lenore S. Powell, Ed.D and Katie Courtice. Reading, MA.: Addison Wesley Publishing Company, 1988.

Dementia: A Practical Guide to Alzheimer's Disease and Related Illnesses. Leonard L. Heston, MD and June A. Whitee. New York: W.H. Freeman and Company, 1983.

Helping Families Face Alzheimer's: A Guide for Clergy. Chicago: Alzheimer's Disease and Related Disorders Associates, Inc., 1988.

The 36 Hour Day: A Family Guide to Caring for Persons with Alzheimer's Disease, Relating Dementing Illness and Memory Loss in Later Life. Nancy L. Mace and Peter V. Rabins, MD. Baltimore: Johns Hopkins University Press, 1981.

Understanding Alzheimer's Disease: What It is, How to Cope with it, Future Directions. Edited by Miriam K. Aronson, Ed. D. Alzheimer's Disease and Related Disorders Association. New York: Charles Scribner's Sons, 1988.

When Your Loved One Has Alzheimer's: A Caregiver's Guide. David L. Carroll. New York: Harper and Row, 1989.

Resources

To find more information and a support group near you, contact:

> Alzheimer's Disease and Related Disorders
> Associates, Inc.
> 70 East Lake Street, Suite 600
> Chicago, IL 60601
> 1-800-621-0379 (excluding Illinois)
> 1-800-572-6037 (for Illinois)

Joan D. Roberts is a pseudonym for the author, who writes from Ohio.